Hello Beautiful Skin!

A Resource on How to Get Rid of Warts, Moles and Skin
Lesions Naturally or with Professional Help

By: Elizabeth Reynolds

9781681275192

PUBLISHERS NOTES

Disclaimer – Speedy Publishing LLC

This publication is intended to provide helpful and informative material. It is not intended to diagnose, treat, cure, or prevent any health problem or condition, nor is intended to replace the advice of a physician. No action should be taken solely on the contents of this book. Always consult your physician or qualified health-care professional on any matters regarding your health and before adopting any suggestions in this book or drawing inferences from it.

The author and publisher specifically disclaim all responsibility for any liability, loss or risk, personal or otherwise, which is incurred as a consequence, directly or indirectly, from the use or application of any contents of this book.

Any and all product names referenced within this book are the trademarks of their respective owners. None of these owners have sponsored, authorized, endorsed, or approved this book.

Always read all information provided by the manufacturers' product labels before using their products. The author and publisher are not responsible for claims made by manufacturers.

This book was originally printed before 2014. This is an adapted reprint by Speedy Publishing LLC with newly updated content designed to help readers with much more accurate and timely information and data.

Speedy Publishing LLC

40 E Main Street, Newark, Delaware, 19711

Contact Us: 1-888-248-4521

Website: http://www.speedypublishing.co

REPRINTED Paperback Edition: 9781681275192:

Manufactured in the United States of America

DEDICATION

This book is dedicated to my friend and soon-to-be-husband, Johnny. You mean the world to me. Thank you for accepting me – flaws and all.

TABLE OF CONTENTS

Chapter 1 - The Truth Behind Warts

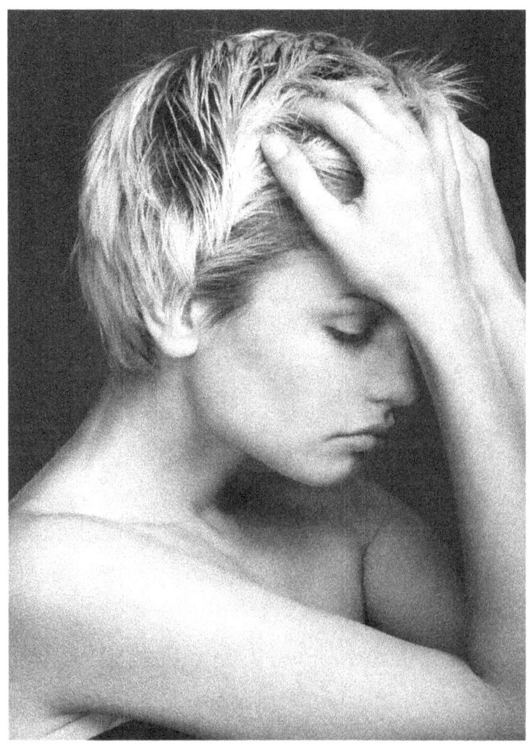

Let's begin by getting rid of one old wives tale. Warts are not caused by coming into contact with frogs or toads! Despite the fact that these creatures have notoriously 'warty' skin, the condition in humans is nothing to do with either frogs or toads! Warts are actually caused by a viral infection, and are known to be benign tumors in the epidermal layer of the skin.

The virus that causes warts is known as the human papilloma virus (or HPV for short) which is a double-stranded DNA virus that causes warts to develop in the outer layers of the skin when it enters the body through a cut or abrasion. Once the virus has gained access to the body, it remains in the inner or lower layers of the epidermis where it may remain totally unnoticed and benign. If it does not do so, however, you get warts developing.

There are many different types of HPV, and there are therefore many different types of warts that can develop in different parts of the human body. Generally speaking, warts are not dangerous, although it is known that some strains of HPV can be responsible for causing cervical and other related cancers. Warts are common and most people are likely to find warts on their skin at least once during the course of their lifetime.

In general, they are nothing more than unsightly and troublesome, but they can occasionally become painful if, for example they were to appear on the heel of your foot, making it difficult and uncomfortable to walk. In addition to the old wives tale about warts being caused by frogs, people also often believe that warts have 'roots', whereas in fact they do not. Warts go no deeper than the top layers of the skin because the human papilloma virus can penetrate no deeper into the body than this.

It is common for warts to feel hard on the outside, and sometimes even perhaps a little abrasive. However, this hardness only comes about as a direct result of contact with the outside air, and wart itself is soft and pliable in its natural state. As a general rule, warts tend to grow as cylindrical columns that issue upwards and outwards from the skin. These tiny cylindrical columns will usually fuse together to cause what you would recognize as a wart, although this is less common when the wart is on the face, because the thinness of the skin in this area of the body prevents this from happening. However, when the wart is growing on a part of your body where the skin is thicker, like your fingers or hands, the individual cylindrical columns will fuse together to become the tightly packed mass of what you would recognize as a wart.

Most commonly, when a wart grows in a part of the body where the skin is thicker, the surface will have a mosaic pattern which is sometimes broken up by black dots. These are actually the visible broken ends of blood vessels which grow quickly but irregularly into a wart. Warts need a blood flow to survive, so if you attempt to cut a wart out, you should expect to bleed, often quite profusely.

The Different Wart-Causing Viruses

According to Wikipedia, there are around 130 different strains of HPV, a proportion of which cause several types of warts. Others are known to cause cancer, while there are strains of HPV that appear to have little or no effect. Everyone who is infected by HPV will react differently to other people simply because every human being is different. Indeed, at any given moment, there are probably millions of people all over the world who have been infected with one strain of HPV or another who are not going to develop any kind of wart problem.

While the most common types of warts tend to develop on the fingers and hands, it is possible for different kind of warts to develop anywhere on the body, including the genital and rectal area, and even inside the mouth. The exact cause of human papilloma virus is unknown, hence it is not possible to protect against or minimize the risk of infection from the virus.

Consequently, while doctors know how to treat warts once they appear, there is little that they can do to prevent those warts appearing, although it is possible to be screened for HPV. Because there are so many different strains of HPV, there are also many different types of warts. Not all of these warts can be treated in exactly the same way. For example, while some types of wart can be treated with over the counter medicines and got rid of within a few days, there are others that can take months to get rid of (if you can get rid of them at all).

Hello Beautiful Skin!

It is also common for a wart that has been removed to grow back in the same place, but because the returning wart may not necessarily be caused by exactly the same strain of HPV, the treatment for it could be entirely different the second time around. Some warts can be extremely painful, while others are totally benign and almost unnoticed.

In the latter situation, and particularly if the wart is in a place where it will not be seen, many people would probably choose to leave the wart well alone. In this situation, it becomes a matter of personal choice and taste with there being no great need to do anything about getting rid of the offending wart.

Facts that You Must Know

1. It is children and teenagers who are most susceptible to warts, with many experts suggesting that one in every ten children or teenagers will suffer warts.

2. Warts are extremely contagious, with the most common cause of infection being direct contact with another wart sufferer. However, the infection can also be spread by contact with anything carrying the bacteria that cause warts, such as dirty clothing, towels and so on.

3. If you want to avoid warts, practicing good hygiene and staying clean is the primary and easiest way of doing so. In addition, shoes should always be worn in public places if at all possible.

4. If your warts will not go away, you might need to seek the advice and attention of a doctor or dermatologist. Before doing so, however, there are plenty of natural treatments that you can try to use to get rid of your warts yourself (and of course, you are going to read of these treatments in this book).

5. Using home remedies is not generally effective if you are trying to get rid of genital warts. In this situation, medical advice is definitely necessary.

6. Warts are benign tumors that are confined to the epidermal layers of the skin. They occur when the skin cells known as keratinocytes become infected.

Chapter 2- Can I Get Warts By Touching Someone Infected?

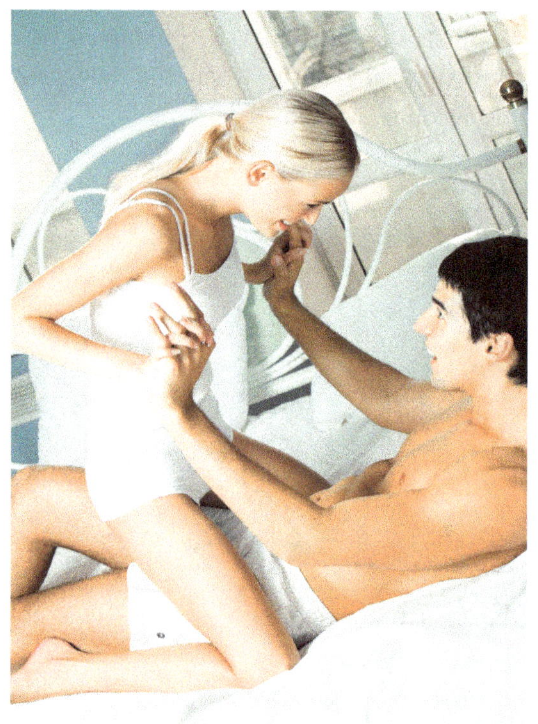

The answer to this question is, yes, warts are highly contagious, although some types of warts are less contagious than others. A wart can be passed from one person to another by nothing more than personal contact. It is even possible to contract warts indirectly by the use of a contaminated towel, for example.

Generally speaking, children tend to contract warts more easily than adults, and because they tend to touch other people more consistently (hugging their parents, for instance), it is from children that the majority of warts are contracted. Most commonly, it is very easy for children to pick up warts on their hands from day-to-day contact with other children who already have warts. This is the most dangerous scenario for the child concerned, because they will often rub their eyes and touch other parts of their body which can very quickly spread the warts.

All kinds of warts are highly contagious, but none more so than genital warts. These are warts that are very easily passed between one sexual partner and the other from vaginal, anal or oral sex. Consequently, if you or your partner is aware that you have genital warts, you must ensure that you only practice safe sex, or that you do not indulge in sexual practices at all. In the case of women who had sex with an infected partner, it is possible to contract genital warts on the cervix.

Genital warts are the number one cause of cervical cancer, and it is possible that a sexually active woman could have warts on her cervix for some time without knowing it. Any woman who suspects that her sexual partner has genital warts should seek medical advice as soon as possible.

The bottom line is, the only way of preventing warts is by adopting very high levels of cleanliness and hygiene at all times. For example, if someone in the family has warts, you should make certain that they use their own towels and that these are changed regularly.

Who is Most Susceptible for Wart Infections?

Children are especially prone to warts, as are teenagers. However, irrespective of age or gender, anyone, anywhere can find warts growing on their body. The time that it takes for a wart to develop will vary from person to person. Some people might find a wart developing on their body almost immediately after coming in contact with an infected person, while some people will never have a wart problem because their natural immune system has the ability to protect them against HPV.

Once you have a wart, it is possible that it will go away entirely naturally in as little as a couple of weeks, while on the other hand, some warts can hang around for many months or even years and be extremely difficult to get rid of. Yet again, it comes down to the individual wart sufferer. If you have a strong, healthy immune system, it will generally make it far more likely that your body will naturally 'solve' your wart problem, but it does not always follow.

What is more likely is that if you have an immune system that has been weakened by a pre-existing medical condition like AIDS or something as invasive as chemotherapy, it becomes far easier for warts to develop.

Furthermore, it is probably going to be far more difficult to get rid of them as well simply because your body would be far less capable of 'fighting back' when your immune system is weakened or otherwise compromised.

Chapter 3- What Kind of Wart Do You Have?

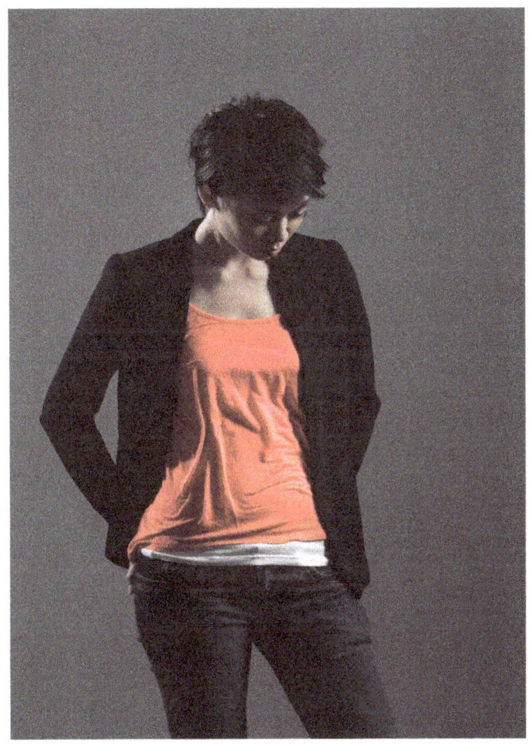

There are several different types of warts. The common wart is the one you would most often find on your hands and fingers. There are also plantar warts or foot warts which can be found on the soles of the feet, normally under the surface of the skin. Depending on where they are located, these can have a debilitating impact on a person's ability to walk.

Flat warts are flat on their surface and often grouped in large numbers. They can be found on the legs, of adult females mostly, or the faces of small children.

Genital warts are one of the most common sexually-transmitted diseases (STD) out there, and treated differently, for the most part, than the other classifications of warts. Although there are several common ways warts are dealt with, Genital warts should not be treated with any of these methods. They could cause you serious harm and damage. Please reserve these common remedies only to warts on your feet, hands, legs and other non-genital regions. If you want to treat genital warts, your best bet is to consult with your doctor.

Some warts will eventually go away on their own, although doctors do not seem to know why this happens. It may take months or years, but some warts simply disappear one day never to be seen again. Others require treatment to deal with them and make them go away.

Even if a wart is not causing you physical pain or discomfort, it is a good idea to look at treating them. Just having the warts can allow them to spread and infect other parts of your body as well as infect other people.

Kind of Wart per HPV Strain

As there are many different strains of HPV, it logically follows that there are many different types of warts as well.

Most of the virus strains shown are harmless, but there are a few of the strains which are mentioned which are generally considered to pose a serious health risk:

And to present some perspective on how likely it is that cervical cancer could result from an HPV infection, this chart gives a clear indication of how many cancer cases are believed to be caused by HPV infection on an annual basis:

As you can see, it is suggested that almost all cervical cancer cases result from HPV infection. Hence, it is absolutely essential that any woman who has any reason to suspect that she might have contracted warts through unsafe sex with an infected partner must seek professional medical attention as soon as possible.

Let us therefore look at some of the more common type of warts, starting with…

Common or Classic Warts

Common or classic warts are most commonly found on the hands and feet, but they can also develop in other areas of the body such as the knees or elbows. Typically, the uppermost surface of a common wart will be raised above the surrounding skin and will present a mosaic or cauliflower like appearance. Generally speaking, common warts are not painful nor do they present any particular danger to the sufferer. Nevertheless, most people would consider these warts to be unpleasant and unsightly, meaning that they want to get rid of common warts if at all possible.

Plantar Warts

Plantar warts (commonly known as a verruca) are typically found on the soles of the feet, especially at pressure points such as on the heels or balls of the feet. While these warts are not particularly dangerous, they can be very painful because of the fact that they grow inwards. Plantar warts can often be mistaken for corns or calluses, but they are recognizable because they are generally flesh colored growths that are hard, flat and have very clearly defined boundaries.

Under normal circumstances, plantar warts will show the small black dots caused by broken blood vessel ends which would give you a further indication that you have plantar warts, rather than corns or calluses. Because they are generally found at pressure points on the soles of the feet, these warts can be extremely painful.

Consequently, as children in particular are very prone to plantar warts, it is often the case that the warts mean they can hardly walk at all. Compared to many other types of wart, plantar warts are not especially contagious, but the particular strain of HPV that causes them thrives in moist, warm conditions like those that would be found in locker rooms or public swimming pools. It is for this reason that plantar warts are very common in youngsters who use public swimming pools on a regular basis.

Extended time in the water softens the soles of their feet, the abrasive edge of the pool cuts or scratches their feet, and finally they enter the communal changing area. In these circumstances, it is hardly any wonder that so many children who enjoy swimming end up with warts almost every time they go to the public pool.

It is possible for plantar warts to disappear entirely naturally, but it is far more likely that they will spread if left untreated. For this reason, it is always best to treat plantar warts as soon after discovery as possible, because if they are left untreated, they can grow to an inch or more. Furthermore, because they shed infectious cells all over the sole of the foot very quickly, it does not take long for a community of plantar warts to develop if the initial infection is not quickly dealt with.

The situation is further complicated by the fact that plantar warts can be extremely painful, so there is no question but that the wart has to be dealt with immediately. Although there is a chance that it might go away on its own (depending on the strength of your immune system), it is pretty unlikely, and who wants to wait while they are in pain?

Periungual or Subungual Warts

These are warts that appear around the nails of both the fingers and toes, causing roughening of the skin surface and some peeling. In order for warts to develop, there must be some existing damage to the skin around the nail, including the situation where shards of the nail break off at the sides, where the skin is damaged at the base of the nail or where the nails have been cut too short.

Warts of this type appear raised and uneven, plus they can cause damage to the nail itself by separating it from the skin or causing the nail to partially detach. If the wart spreads under the nail, the pressure generated by the growth of the wart can cause considerable pain and in a worst-case scenario, if the wart causes damage to the nail matrix, a deformed nail structure could be the final result.

It is generally suggested that periungual warts can be more difficult than most other types to get rid of, and they will often be accompanied by unpleasant symptoms such as itching (very commonly) or pain (less so). Whether it is itching or pain, both of these symptoms would make it extremely likely that anyone suffering from periungual or subungual warts would definitely want to do something to improve their condition as quickly as possible.

Flat Warts

Many people who have flat warts do not even know that they have them. This is because the most common flat warts that people are actually aware of are brown marks on the skin that they treat as 'sun spots' or even beauty spots! Flat warts of this nature will generally appear as a result of too much exposure to the sun. Sunshine 'activates' the particular strain of human papilloma virus that causes flat warts to become active. In effect, the virus has been underneath the skin for some time and has remained 'dormant' but the necessary 'dose' of sunlight has triggered a reaction.

This particular variety of wart might be brown (as suggested), but is not necessarily so because you will sometimes see them in a variety of colors including white, pink and yellow. While many flat warts do not protrude above skin level (hence the name), some may do so and they can sometimes 'rise' to a slight point.

Generally speaking, flat warts are unlikely to cause pain or discomfort and can appear on the face, back of the neck, legs, arms and hands. They are very commonly seen in children who spend a lot of their time acquiring the cuts and scratches that are necessary for the HPV strain 3 or 10 to infect the body.

Genital Warts

This is the name that is applied to warts that men suffer in the groin or on the penis. Most commonly, genital warts come up in clusters and are clearly visible. Given that they are most commonly passed from one sexual partner to another during unprotected sex, the simple way of ensuring that warts of this nature do not occur is to avoid sexual encounters with those who have them. As suggested previously, it is possible for genital warts to infect both sexes, with the female version being known as 'vaginal warts'.

A third variation is anal warts which are small clusters of the same warts that appear around the anal hole which are once again sexually transmitted. However, in the same way that vaginal warts may not be visible if they have infected the cervix, so anal warts may be invisible if they are only present inside the anus.

Another important consideration is that genital, vaginal or anal warts do not have to be visible for any individual to be a carrier of the HPV virus. Hence, it is possible that you could be infected by someone who has no outward signs of infection if you are not practicing safe sex (or abstaining).

According to the statistics reported by Wikipedia, it is believed that HPV is the most commonly contracted sexually transmitted disease in the USA. In fact, it is estimated that 75-80% of sexually active Americans will contract HPV at some time in their life while the Center for Disease Control (CDC) suggests that some 80% of US woman will have contracted at least one strain of HPV before they reach age 50.

Given all of these statistics and suggestions, there can be little doubt that the chances of being infected with one of the HPV strains that cause anogenital warts (between them, HPV strains 6 and 11 are responsible for 90% of cases) is remarkably high. There can therefore be no argument against the suggestion that anyone suffering from warts of this nature should do whatever is necessary to prevent them infecting other people.

However, it is important to understand that home remedies are not appropriate for the treatment of genital warts. While there are various products that are claimed to get rid of genital warts completely naturally, it is still probably the best idea to seek medical attention if you have any reason to suspect that you have been infected with HPV.

Chapter 4- Wart Treatments that You Can Do at Home

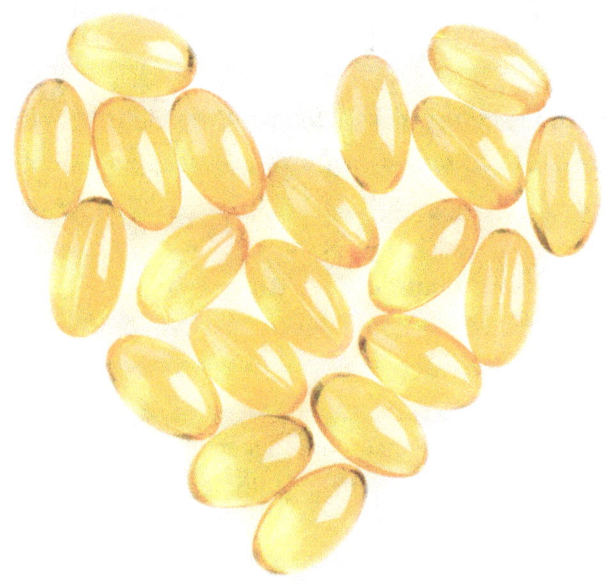

There are plenty of different natural home remedies that people use every day to get rid of warts. However, not every wart removal method will be as effective for everyone because every individual reacts differently to various treatment methods. However, some or all of the following entirely natural wart treatments might work for you, and there is definitely no harm in trying to use any or all of these natural treatment strategies before turning to pharmaceutical drug–based treatments.

The Duct Tape Method

It is generally believed that using duct tape to get rid of warts is effective in up to 80% of cases, so as strange as it may sound, it is definitely worth trying duct tape as your first wart removal option of choice. The method involves nothing more than placing a small piece of duct tape on the wart, thus sealing the wart in an airless 'tomb'. Whether it is this ability to seal the wart (denying it the ability to 'breathe') that makes it effective or whether there is some acid in the adhesive used on this particular type of tape that kills the wart is still open to debate, but the fact is, it works.

In fact, when this method of getting rid of warts was the first posited by Dr. Anthony J. Mancini (head of dermatology at the Children's Memorial Hospital in Chicago), it was discovered that it was (and still is) every bit as effective as far more expensive treatment methods such as cryotherapy, so it is definitely worth trying. Using duct tape, you cover the wart with tape and leave it covered (replace the tape as necessary) for six or seven days, after which time you should start to see some results.

Whether there is any evidence of progress after this time period or not, you should remove the tape and soak the wart so that it becomes soft and malleable. You should apply a pumice stone or an emery board to scrub or scratch off the upper levels of the wart. After this, you reapply the tape for another week and do the same again.

Removing a wart using the duct tape method can take several weeks, but it is extremely popular because it is simple, cheap and entirely natural. However, because it is possible for your body to get rid of a wart in the time it takes for the duct tape method to be effective; it can be a little difficult to know for sure whether it is your body's natural reaction or the duct tape that removes the wart. Nevertheless, because as many as four out of every five people who use this method of removal can find it effective, it is worth a go.

Banana Skins

Applying the inside of banana skins to your warts is also believed to help to get rid of warts. In this case, it is believed that the slightly acidic nature of the inside of the banana skin helps to cauterize the warts away. Apply a small piece of the banana skin to the wart and tape it in place, because once again, it needs to be left in contact with the wart for several days before any beneficial effects are likely to be noticed.

If the wart that you are trying to get rid of is in a highly visible place, you are probably going to feel a little foolish walking around with a piece of banana skin taped to your body. Consequently, this is a wart treatment strategy that works best if you apply the banana skin shortly before retiring to bed and leaving it in place overnight.

Salicylic Acid

Salicylic acid is an acid that is extracted from the bark of the willow tree, and is yet another solution that is used to 'burn' warts away. Using salicylic acid based product to get rid of your warts does require a good deal more attention and action because the solution needs applying once or twice every day.

On the other hand, using a salicylic acid based treatment is likely to get rid of your warts more quickly than either of the two previous treatment methods, so for this reason; it is a treatment method that is extremely popular.

Depending on the kind of wart that you are treating with salicylic acid, the experts suggest that a different strength of solution should be used. However, there is some disagreement about exactly what solution strength is most effective in specific cases.

For instance, if you are using it to deal with plantar warts, then there are websites that suggest that the salicylic solution needs to be at least 40% acid. On the other hand, there are other sites where it is suggested that a solution of only 15% acid will be strong enough to get rid of exactly the same type of warts. Consequently, it is a little difficult to know exactly what strength of acid solution to use.

Even though salicylic acid is a natural substance, it is nevertheless still an acid. For this reason, I would recommend using the weakest solution possible to start with to see how effective it is. Only if you discover that it is not working should you move to using a stronger solution. Salicylic acid will be most effective if the area to be treated has been properly prepared. It should be soaked in warm water to make it soft, before removing the top layer of wart skin with an abrasive such as an emery board.

Apply the solution as directed, and then cover the wart with a band aid as it encourages the absorption of the acid solution. Many of the best known over-the-counter wart treatments such as Compound W. and Clear Away use salicylic acid as the primary active ingredient. It is also possible to buy acid based products on the internet, as you have already seen from previous screen shots.

It is necessary to use care when applying salicylic acid so that you do not apply it to healthy skin surrounding the wart. While it is unlikely to do any serious or long-lasting damage, it can nevertheless be irritating, causing itching and redness.

Hello Beautiful Skin!
Aloe Vera

Aloe Vera is something of a 'wonder' treatment, because irrespective of what kind of skin problem you have, aloe vera will probably help, and warts are no exception to this. In order to treat warts using aloe vera, the best thing to do is use aloe vera juice, and while it is possible to grow your own aloe vera plants, it is not at all easy to extract the juice effectively. For this reason, it makes sense to treat you warts with aloe vera juice that has been commercially extracted, or to use an aloe vera based cream. Whichever way you do it, soak a cotton ball in the aloe vera solution, and apply it to the wart.

Use a Band-Aid or a strip of medical tape to keep the cotton ball in place, and re-soak it in the aloe vera solution as necessary. Continue to wear the band aid and cotton ball combination in direct contact with the wart for several days, and you should start to see some positive results fairly quickly.

Tea Tree Oil

Tea tree oil is an essential oil produced from the Melaleuca alternifolia tree which is a native shrub found in Northern Australia. Tea tree oil is acknowledged to be a strong antifungal and antibiotic agent with well-known antiseptic qualities. Because of its ability to kill almost any bacteria, it is an extremely popular way of getting rid of warts which have grown on the skin as a direct result of HPV bacterial infection.

Application of tea tree oil to warts could not be simpler. Unlike using aloe vera, there is no need for cotton balls or Band-Aids, because all that is needed is a daily application of the oil to the offending wart to start seeing positive results in just a few days.

Indeed, if anything, tea tree oil is even more effective than aloe vera for getting rid of warts completely naturally.

The rate of successful wart removal from tea tree oil application is high, so using tea tree oil to get rid of warts is one of the most popular natural treatment methods.

Castor Oil

Castor oil is derived from the Ricinus communis plant which contains undecylenic acid, a powerful dermal antifungal that once again attacks warts at the bacterial level. The acid is the active ingredient in many over-the-counter skin treatments as it is highly effective for relieving itching, burning and other common skin irritations. Not only does undecylenic acid have antifungal qualities, it is also known to have antiviral and antibacterial qualities, hence its effectiveness as a natural wart treatment.

Echinacea

Echinacea is a popular herbal remedy that is extracted from the purple cone flower that is indigenous to North America. For many centuries, it was used as a treatment by the Plains Indians of North America for a wide range of medical complaints due to its general medicinal qualities, primarily its ability to boost the strength of the immune system and to help ward off viral infections. While it is primarily viewed as a treatment for warding off winter conditions like colds and flu, it is also a natural antibiotic which is therefore effective for treating infections and fighting off bacteria.

Since having a strong and healthy immune system is the key to your body being able to get rid of warts without any additional interventional treatment, the fact that echinecea is known to boost that system is an extremely good reason for taking Echinacea in either tablet or extract form.

Vitamin E Oil and Garlic

Vitamin E (which is generally obtained from vegetable oil) is believed to be a powerful antioxidant and helps get rid of warts because of these qualities. It helps to promote skin regeneration so it is also highly effective for preventing scarring after a wart has been removed. In addition, garlic is believed to buoy up the immune system, meaning that taking garlic capsules is likely to make your body far more resistant to warts than it would otherwise be. Combining this with applying vitamin E oil to your warts is a twin pronged attack that should be effective.

Other Homemade Remedies

1. Apple Cider Vinegar: Saturate a cotton ball with apple cider vinegar (ACV) and apply to wart, secure in place with a Band-Aid or tape. Do this every night before bed, remove in the morning. Good for all warts, recommended especially for Plantar and flat warts.

2. White Household Vinegar & Baking Soda: Sprinkle a heavy coat of baking soda on the wart then drizzle vinegar over it. Do this once in the morning and once at night until wart is gone.

3. Baking Soda: Make a thick paste of baking soda and water, apply to wart and cover with tape or a Band-Aid.

4. Clear Nail Polish: Paint the wart with a coat of clear nail polish; reapply as needed until wart is gone.

5. Hydrogen Peroxide: Apply to wart each day using a cotton swab.

6. Toothpaste: Dab regular toothpaste generously on top of the wart then cover with a Band-Aid. Do this daily until wart is gone.

7. Aspirin: Rub wart with olive oil then place an aspirin tablet on top and secure with a piece of tape or Band-Aid. Change daily. Or crush an aspirin tablet fine then add a few drops of water to make a paste. Apply to wart and cover with a Band-Aid. Watch on sensitive skin.

8. Vitamin C Tablet: Crush the Vitamin C tablet fine then make a paste with water. Apply to wart and wrap it with tape or a Band-Aid to secure. Change daily.

Try Fruits and Vegetables Too!

1. Potatoes: Cut a potato in half and rub the potato juice over the wart.

2. Lemons: Rub a slice of lemon over the wart for 5 minutes twice a day. You can also dab lemon juice directly on the wart.

3. Limes: Rub a slice of freshly cut lime over the wart for 5 minutes twice a day. You can also dab lime juice directly on the wart.

4. Eggplant: Cut a thin slice of eggplant just a bit larger than the wart and hold in place with a piece of tape or Band-Aid. Change daily until wart has disappeared. Good remedy for children or those with sensitive skin.

5. Onion: Rub a slice of freshly cut onion over the wart twice a day. You can also sprinkle onion slice with salt first then apply to wart. Another suggested treatment is to drizzle lemon juice on the wart then cover with a freshly cut piece of onion (wrap a piece of tape or Band-Aid around to hold in place).

6. Carrots: Grate a fresh carrot then mix with olive oil until you have a thick paste. Apply to wart and cover with a Band-Aid. Do this twice a day until wart disappears.

7. Apples: Apply a freshly cut slice of apple to the wart and secure in place with tape or a Band-Aid. Change twice a day until wart is gone.

8. Figs: Mix mashed fig with a bit of olive oil and apply to wart, cover with a Band-Aid. Do this daily until wart is gone.

9. Radishes: Cut a slice of radish just the size of the wart, cover the wart and secure in place with a Band-Aid. Change daily.

10. Pineapple: Apply a freshly cut piece of pineapple to the wart morning, noon and night until wart is gone.

Oils and Extracts

1. Witch Hazel: Rub Witch Hazel into the wart a couple times a day.

2. Clove Oil: Mix a few drops of clove oil with olive oil then apply to wart, change daily.

3. Grapefruit Seed Extract: Apply a few drops to the pad of a Band-Aid then cover wart, change daily.

4. Oil of Oregano: Mix a few drops with olive oil then apply to the pad of a Band-Aid–cover wart and change daily.

5. Lavender Essential Oil: Carefully dab the wart with a drop of Lavender EO, cover with a Band-Aid. Do this once a day.

6. Geranium Essential Oil: Mix a few drops with olive oil then apply to the pad of a Band-Aid–cover wart and change daily.

7. Lemon Essential Oil: Mix a few drops with olive oil then apply to the pad of a Band-Aid–cover wart and change daily.

8. Frankincense: Apply a drop directly to the wart and cover with tape or a Band-Aid. Change Band-Aid daily. Reapply drop of Frankincense twice a week.

9. Vegetable Oil: Smother the wart with a thick coat of vegetable oil then apply tape or a bandage. Do this each night before bed and first thing in the morning.

Herbs and Plants

1. Dandelions: Apply dandelion milk from the stem of a dandelion to the wart. Cover with tape or a Band-Aid. Apply two times a day until wart is removed.

2. Basil Leaves: Crush fresh basil leaves and cover the wart then secure in place with a Band-Aid.

3. Marigolds: Break open marigold leaves and apply the plant juice directly to wart. Do this daily until wart is gone.

4. Milkweed: A Native American wart remedy is to rub the milk from a milkweed plant into the wart several times a day until wart has been removed.

Commercially Produced Natural Wart Treatments

There are quite a number of websites from where you can buy natural wart treatments, many of which contain a mixture of some of the natural treatments that we have already considered in this report. For example, both Naturasil Extra Strength and Dermisil base their products on a combination of tea tree and castor oils.

There are many other natural wart cure products that you can buy either online or across the counter in your local high street or shopping mall. However, be aware that many products do not list the ingredients that they use, which means that you have no way of knowing for certain just how natural those products really are.

Consequently, if you are looking at a product where you have no information about the ingredients, you will have to make your own decision about whether you are satisfied that the product is entirely natural or not.

Chapter 5- Wart Treatments Administered by Professionals

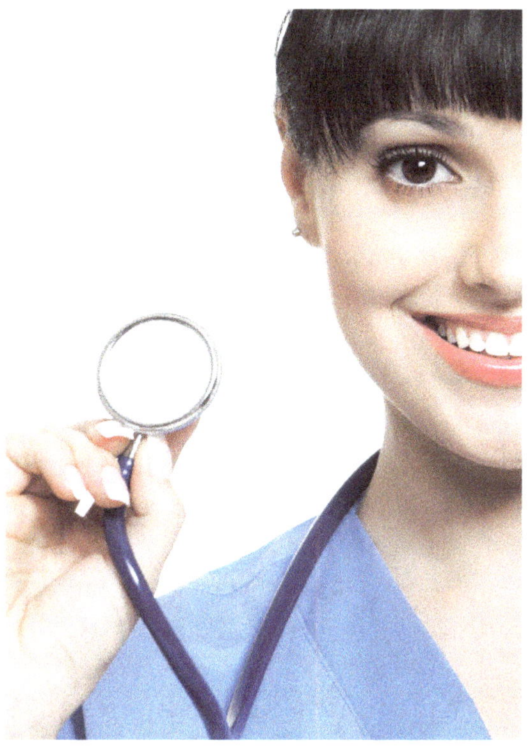

If you have stubborn warts and home treatment isn't helping, your doctor may suggest one of the following approaches, based on the location of your wart, the degree of your symptoms and your preferences. Doctors generally start with the least painful, least destructive methods, especially in young children.

Acid: One of the most common methods is to burn warts off with a mild acid applied topically to the wart. Many applications may be required over the course of several weeks to achieve this. Salicylic acid, cantharidin, and dichloroacetic (or trichloroacetic) acid are useful. Removing a wart with salicylic acid can be done by cleaning the area, applying the acid, and removing the dead skin with a pumice stone or emery board. It may take up to 50 weeks to remove a wart. Other acid methods may be used.

Cryotherapy

Cryotherapy or freezing warts is generally considered to be one of the most effective natural wart treatments, but it does not come without its 'costs'.

Firstly, it costs considerably more to use cryotherapy to get rid of your warts than it would if you get rid of them using something as simple as duct tape or banana skins. Secondly, the process involves using a substance like liquid nitrogen to freeze the wart and also the skin around it. While the application of liquid nitrogen using a spray or a cotton swab generally takes less than a minute, it can be quite a painful way of having your warts removed. Consequently, cryotherapy is generally administered by your healthcare professional and they will in some circumstances use a local anesthetic, particularly if requested to do so.

Furthermore, pain from cryotherapy can last up to three days, and it may be necessary to undergo treatment several times in order to get rid of the wart completely. This is because freezing it in this way tends to kill only the top of the wart, so you may require as many as four cryotherapy sessions (spread one to three weeks apart) to finally get rid of more persistent warts. Within hours of undergoing treatment, you may find that a blister forms.

When this happens, it is common for the blister to burst, in which case you should immediately clean and disinfect the area in order to stop the spread of the wart virus. You should avoid contact with the fluid emanating from the blister as this may be carrying the virus as well. The blister will dry up over the course of the next few days, and it may well be that the wart falls off as part of the same process.

So, the crucial question is, how effective is cryotherapy for getting rid of warts? It is generally believed that it will be effective in between 35- 65% of cases, but that it is no more effective than using salicylic acid, and even the duct tape method is likely to be every bit as effective as cryotherapy (if not more so). So, the conclusion about cryotherapy must be, it might work but there are certainly other things that you should try before resorting to using liquid nitrogen to freeze off your warts.

Incidentally, it is now possible to buy liquid nitrogen across the pharmacy or drug store counter to treat you at home, but before being tempted to do so, there are other natural treatments that are far less expensive and painful.

Cantharidin

Cantharidin is a poisonous chemical compound that is secreted by the male of many different types of blister beetle, particularly Lytta vesicatoria, or the Spanish fly as it is more commonly known. The first thing to note about using cantharidin is that it is definitely not something to be ingested, because as little as 10 mg of it is potentially fatal. However, when it is diluted, cantharidin is highly effective for removing warts because it is a powerful blistering agent that literally 'burns' the wart out because it is so strongly caustic.

Generally speaking, at the time of application (either something that you do for yourself, or something that your doctor might do), there will be no pain or discomfort. However, once the wart starts blistering anything between three and eight hours later, some discomfort or pain might be felt. After application of cantharidin, you should cover the wart with a Band-Aid or bandage as appropriate and remove it again 24 hours later. At that point, you (or your doctor) should remove as much of the wart as possible (with the emery board, pumice stone or by 'slicing off' the top layer of warty skin).

Given that one application of cantharidin is often enough to get rid of warts once and for all, this will often mean removing what little is left! Sometimes, the treatment is not 100% successful the first time, and it might therefore be that you need to apply cantharidin again in order to banish the wart completely.

Minor Surgery

This involves cutting away the wart tissue or destroying it by using an electric needle in a process called electrodessication and curettage. However, the injection of anesthetic given before this surgery can be painful, and the surgery may leave a scar. For these reasons, surgery is usually reserved for warts that haven't responded to other therapies. Note: The excision of warts is not recommended since the surgery may leave a painful scar and it is common for warts to return in the scar tissue.

Laser Surgery

Laser surgery can be expensive, and it may leave a scar. It's usually reserved for tough-to-treat warts. New technology has enabled doctors to use lasers to destroy the wart. The procedure, performed in the physician's office, is expensive and is likely to result in some scarring. Its efficacy in comparison to other destructive approaches in unproven.

Medicines Prescribed by Doctors

If you have a bad case of warts that hasn't responded to standard treatments, your doctor may refer you to a dermatologist for further treatment, including:

Immunotherapy

This type of treatment attempts to harness your body's natural rejection system to fight off warts. Topical immunotherapy medications that may be prescribed for stubborn warts include squaric acid dibutylester and a gel called imiquimod (Aldara). Imiquimod is marketed for the treatment of genital warts but has also proved effective for treating common warts. However, warts may return when these therapies are stopped.

Bleomycin (Blenoxane)

Your doctor may inject a wart with a medication called Bleomycin, which kills the virus. Bleomycin is used with caution for warts, but in higher doses, is used to treat some kinds of cancer. Risks of this therapy include nail loss and damage to the skin and nerves.

Retinoids

Derived from vitamin A, these medications disrupt your wart's skin cell growth. Your doctor may prescribe a retinoid cream or an oral medication. These medications make your skin extra sensitive to the sun, so be sure to protect your skin from the sun while taking them.

Common warts can be tough to get rid of completely or permanently, especially when they appear around and under your nails. And, if you're susceptible to the wart virus, you probably always will be. New warts may crop up even after a successful treatment. More than one treatment may be necessary to manage the problem. Warts are viral, and antibiotics are not effective for viral illnesses.

There are many other treatments available for the treatment of warts. No single therapy is so effective that it has eliminated the use of all others. Ultimately, all treatments rely on the patient's immune system to recognize the wart virus proteins and to produce an immune response that will rid the body of this annoying problem.

Chapter 6- Other Possible Wart Treatments

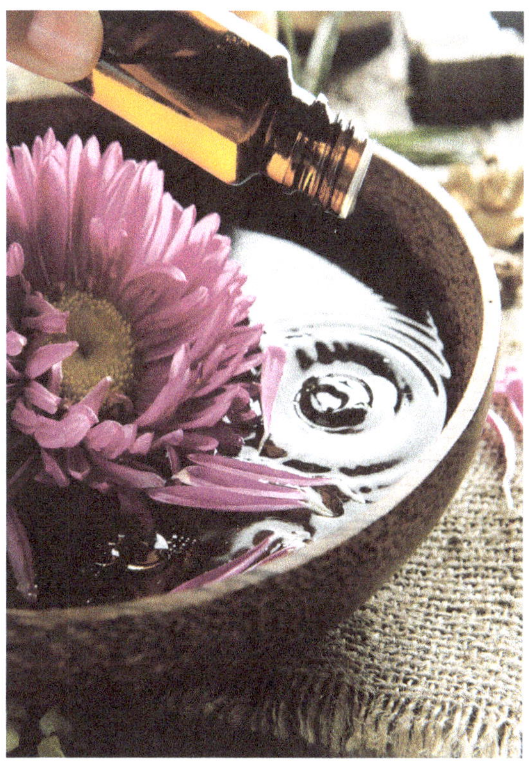

Wart Soaks

Soaking the warts daily in treated baths will help soften them and help the warts respond to treatment. Can also help fight the virus and prevent infection. Soaking treatments are also worthwhile doing before sloughing the skin with an emery board or pumice stone. Soak wart daily in a warm bath of baking soda and water.

1. Soak wart daily in a hot bath of Epsom salt and water.

2. Soak wart in very hot water until it becomes lukewarm (do this daily, don't have the water so hot it burns you though). Plain hot water is fine but you can also add some vinegar.

Hello Beautiful Skin!
Wart Immunity Boosters

Beef up your immunity system so your body can fight the wart virus internally. Here are a few suggested immunity boosters I have on hand that are recommended for fighting warts.

1. Cabbage: Eat a lot of fresh, raw cabbage each day.

2. Garlic: Add fresh, chopped garlic to your food whenever possible. You can also take garlic pills or capsules daily.

3. Limes: Squeeze fresh lime juice over food or add fresh lime juice to a glass of water and drink this twice a day.

4. Broccoli: Eat fresh, raw broccoli daily.

5. Oranges: Eat an orange once a day.

6. Bananas: Good for potassium, eat one a day to fight warts.

7. Onions: Top everything suitable with chopped fresh onion, preferably raw but cooked is fine too.

This information is simply a collection of home remedies for getting rid of warts – not professional medical advice. Please seek a doctor's opinion when unsure or to confirm appropriate treatment for your wart.

CHAPTER 7- MOLES AS SKIN LESIONS

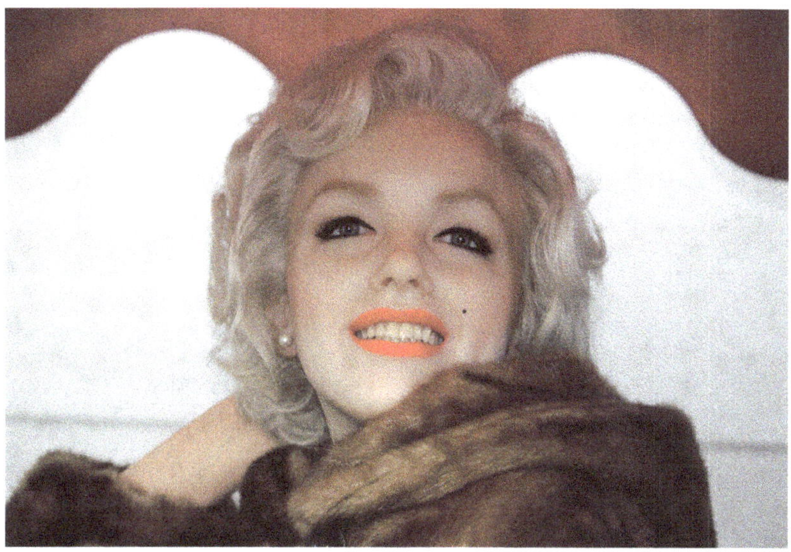

Moles are also lesions of the skin that are medically known as nevi (the singular is nevus), with the word coming from the Latin meaning 'birthmark'. Moles are irregularities of the skin that are formed when cells known as melanocytes grow along with the surrounding skin tissue, clumping together to form a colored mark on the skin.

Generally, a mole will be brown in color, although the color and shape will gradually change over time entirely naturally. Most commonly, this means that the shape changes from a flat macule to a raised papule, with the color gradually changing from brown to that of flesh as the melanocytes migrate from the skin surface to deeper under the skin. This color change will not necessarily be even, sometimes giving the mole a speckled brown appearance that can look somewhat similar to malignant melanomas.

Moles are however totally benign, with the difference between one and the other being clear from a dermatoscopy. Some people are born with moles, but more commonly they grow as a result of exposure to sunlight. Under normal circumstances, it is melanocytes growing in a normal manner that give the skin it's common, natural pigmentation, and it is this 'clumping' effect that creates moles.

Sunlight can encourage this to happen, hence the tendency for moles to occur as a result of extended exposure to the sun. Under normal circumstances, moles are non-cancerous, and although they do change shape and color over time, this is normally a slow process.

Consequently, if a mole changes shape or size quickly, it is best to get it checked with a biopsy. Similarly, if you have a mole that is irregularly shaped, protruding or one that itches or bleeds, you should seek medical advice, as it may possibly be cancerous.

Moles can develop on the skin on their own or in clusters, and they can be found anywhere on the body. While they are most commonly flat or slightly raised above the skin, it is also possible for moles to grow on 'stalks' that are significantly raised above the skin level. In this case, moles that are on stalks will usually fall off of their own accord. Otherwise, in the case of more 'normal' moles, they can be present for up to 50 years before they fall off or begin to fade.

Depending on where they are located, many people find moles to be unsightly and embarrassing. For this reason, they might choose to do whatever is necessary to remove their moles and it is probable that the first course of action they will consider is to visit their doctor to get the job done. However, this is not necessary as there are many effective and completely natural ways of getting rid of moles.

Before considering the different ways of getting rid of moles naturally, let us first consider the etymology of moles in a little more detail.

Who Has Moles?

Moles are extremely common and tend to develop on people between the ages of 10 and 40. Over those years, anyone can develop new moles which might be completely flush with the surface of the skin or slightly raised above it. When moles first appear, they will generally do so as small spots on the skin that gradually expand and are perhaps raised slightly upwards. Over time, moles can change back to their original shape and size with the possibility that the pigmentation will fade and the color will return to that of the surrounding flesh as a direct result.

The majority of people have moles, with the most common age for development being when you are in your late teens and early 20s. This is due the hormonal balance of your body changing at this particular period of life. Any moles that develop around these years will not generally change in shape or size. Because the development of moles can be tied in with hormonal changes, it is common for them to develop at any time in life when the hormonal balance of your body is changing. As an example, it is not unknown for new moles to appear during pregnancy.

However, as previously suggested, moles can be present on the body from birth, as it is believed that up to 3% of newborn babies will already have a least 1 mole on their body. These are almost always noncancerous and totally benign.

The Different Types of Moles

Perhaps surprisingly, there are many different types of moles, with the most common types being junctional, dermal, sebaceous, blue and compound moles. Junctional moles are extremely common, with the majority of them being flat, round and of a dark or light brown hue, perhaps raised slightly off the skin surface. These are the most common moles that the majority of people develop, and they are almost always completely benign.

Dermal moles range in color from that of the surrounding flesh to dark brown, and are often elevated above the skin surface. These are generally found on the upper half of the body (very rarely on the lower half), and will sometimes have a hair growing from them.

Sebaceous moles are usually developed by people who have over-active oil producing glands in the skin, and are always yellow in color. Moles of this type generally have a hard or rough surface, and can sometimes be painful (in which case, seek medical advice).

Blue moles are generally developed by women, although it is not impossible for men to develop them as well. However, the vast majority of blue moles which are developed from natural pigmentation deep inside the skin are seen on the arms, head, face, neck and scalp of women.

Finally, you have compound moles. These are generally raised above the skin and can be of any color, ranging from dark brown to invisible, matching the surrounding flesh perfectly. These moles grow from the deepest layers of the dermis to the upper, outer layers of the skin with the color being dictated by the level of melanocytes present in the mole.

All of these moles are safe, and as a general observation, as long as the shape of the mole is regular and not changing rapidly, you can be fairly confident that there is no danger.

When it's a Mole and When It's Not

If you have a large mole that is of irregular shape and coloring, you should get it checked as soon as possible, because this might suggest that it is a malignant melanoma. Furthermore, people over the age of 50 sometimes develop what is known as lentigomaligna or 'melonotic freckles' as they are sometimes known. These usually appear on the face as a flat, round spot with a tan coloring that can be either consistent (of one shade only) or varied.

Over time, it is likely that the mole will grow darker and larger, and in over 30% of cases, such a mole will turn into lentigo malignant melanoma, which is a skin cancer that can often prove fatal. Hence, this is one type of mole that you should not try to treat naturally.

As a general rule, moles are not dangerous, but if they are painful, irritating or itchy, it is not a good sign and would suggest that you have a problem. In this case, it is always best to seek medical advice as soon as possible, because the natural treatments that you will learn of later are not likely to be suitable for getting rid of any mole or skin lesion that is cancerous (or potentially so).

Also be aware that if a mole grows or rapidly expands, this is another sign that the growth may be malignant. Look for asymmetrical moles too by drawing an imaginary line down the center of your mole and examining either side of it. Both sides should match perfectly otherwise you have an asymmetrical mole which also needs checking as soon as possible. It does not necessarily mean that it is cancerous, but it does mean you should check.

Although the various different moles on your body can be of different shapes and colors (they may be different types of mole after all), each mole should be of a uniform shade. Consequently, if you have a mole that is of two different shades, get it checked out immediately.

Normal moles do not have a noticeable border around them either, whereas a cancerous growth on the skin that might at first appear to be a mole probably will. This border area might also expand and change color as time goes by, once again being suggestive of something that is malignant and therefore in need of immediate medical attention.

CHAPTER 8- MOLE TREATMENTS

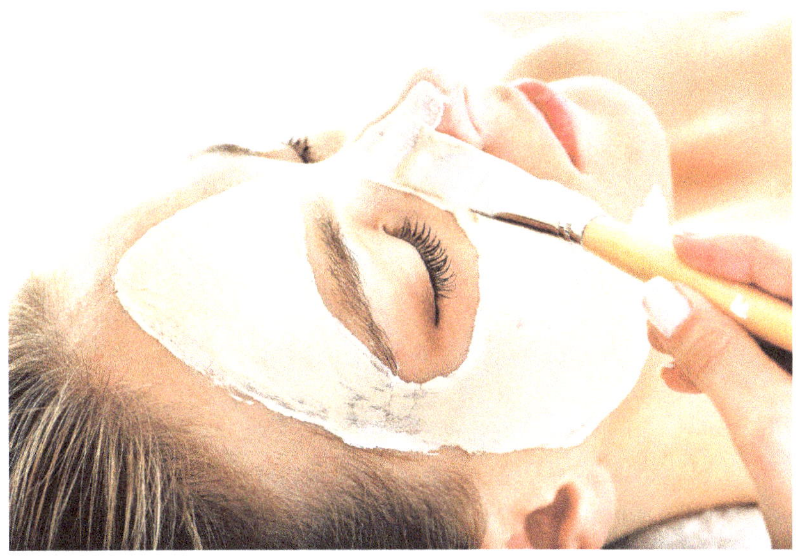

If you are thinking of treating your moles using completely natural methods, you should have a medical checkup before doing so because this will at least confirm that it is safe to use natural remedies. If there is any suspicion that the mole that you want to treat is malignant, your doctor or dermatologist will take appropriate action, but they can also advise you as to whether trying to get rid of your moles naturally is a safe option.

Alternatively, they might suggest that they should treat your moles for you, in which case you should know how they will do so. In some cases, your doctor or dermatologist might suggest that they cut out the mole that you want to get rid of. In this case, they are going to have to cut down into the skin as deep as the mole goes. This could be painful, and depending upon how deep they have to go, it could also leave significant scarring. Scarring is not something you want if you are trying to get rid of the mole because it is unsightly or embarrassing. After all, you would be exchanging the unsightly mole for an equally unsightly scar, which is not appealing especially if it is on your face or neck.

If the mole is only on the surface of the skin, then the procedure necessary for removing it is far less invasive. In this case, your doctor might cauterize the mole off the surface of your skin using a special tool, and because this is only on the surface, there is less likelihood of scarring. Nevertheless, the tool that the doctor uses to cauterize the mole off your skin is potentially capable of causing scarring, so you need to know that the person carrying out the procedure knows what they are doing. For this reason, this is the kind of thing that you're probably best getting done by a dermatologist, rather than by a general medical practitioner who might have limited experience of using the cauterizing tool.

The third and most favored option is for your doctor or dermatologist to use laser therapy to remove your mole, which is particularly common if the mole is highly visible, for example, on your face.

Laser therapy has the major advantage that it is non-invasive and there is no visible wound once the mole has been removed. It is quick, clean and highly effective to use a laser to remove moles, and so if you must use a doctor to get rid of your moles for you, this is undoubtedly the best way of doing so.

Popular Natural Methods for Mole Removal

There are many natural treatments that you can apply to get rid of moles. However, as with natural treatments for warts, not every treatment will work for everyone all of the time. Hence, there is likely to be a degree of trial and error involved when you are using natural methods to get rid of your moles. But as nothing that you are about to read of is in any way invasive or potentially harmful, there is absolutely no reason why you cannot try every one of these remedies until you find one that works for you.

The first method that you could try is to use cauliflower or more specifically, cauliflower juice. Place a quantity of raw cauliflower into your kitchen blender and reduce it to a puree. There is no need to add additional liquids, as there is more than enough water in the cauliflower itself to enable you to do this. Rub the puree on the mole that you want to clear, and you should find that after a week or two the mole will start to peel off your skin naturally.

An alternative method of getting rid of moles is to use garlic. In this case, crush the garlic with the back of a spoon so that you end up with a thick paste-like substance. Put this on to the mole that you want to remove, and cover the area with a band aid or bandage. Apply the garlic paste to the mole every night before going to bed, and remove both the bandage and the paste during the day to allow the mole to breathe. Once again, this should cause the mole to disappear after a couple of weeks.

Pineapple juice is another substance that can help to make moles go away, but it is only effective if you are using freshly squeezed pineapple juice. Juice from a can or a carton is not going to be effective, so you should squeeze fresh juice every day and apply it to the area of skin that you want cleared. Rub the juice onto the affected area on a daily basis, and you should see the offending mole begin to fade and disappear after a couple of weeks.

Instead of pineapple juice, try a combination of castor oil and honey. Between them, these two substances will have a very similar effect to pineapple juice when applied to the area of skin that you want to clear. Try scrubbing the appropriate skin area with extremely hot water five or six times a day, and then apply cider vinegar to the area that you are attempting to treat. Leave the cider vinegar on your skin for 10 to 15 minutes at a time and then rinse it away completely. Do this six or seven times every day for a week or more, and you should see your moles gradually disappear.

The last things that you can try are fig stems. Although these will not necessarily be that easy for many people to find, if you can do so, they are very effective because they contain a juice that is known to be good for removing moles.

As suggested earlier, what is going to be most effective for any individual who is trying to get rid of their moles totally naturally is something that can only be established by trial and error. However, everything you have read of in this section could be effective, so give them a try until you find something that works for you.

Chapter 9- How to Get Rid of Skin Tags

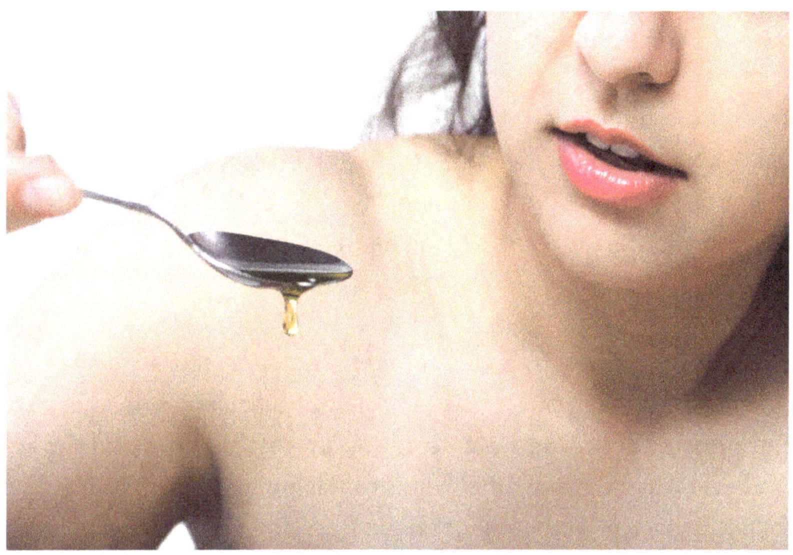

Skin tags are excess folds of skin that dangle from your body. Although these tags are not normally dangerous in any way (they are almost always benign), they are undoubtedly unsightly and the kind of thing that probably makes the skin tag sufferer feel embarrassed. They are usually the same color as the surrounding flesh and are most commonly seen around the neck area, under the arms and even under the breasts. They are most commonly seen when people are advancing in years and are usually the result of continuous rubbing or irritation or a particular part of the body over many years (by clothing, for example).

The most common natural skin tag treatment is to go back to our old friend, the duct tape. Once again, cover the tag with duct tape and leave it until the tape begins to loosen slightly. After it does so, pull the tape away and see if the tag comes with it. If not, keep repeating the process until it does.

Alternatively, try applying vitamin E. oil to the tag and then cover the area with a band aid. Do this two to three times a day and check every time you remove the Band-Aid for whether the tag comes with it. Once again, this is not likely to happen immediately, but keep trying, and eventually it should do.

The third option (and the only one that involves a slight degree of pain) is to 'tie off' the tag so that it is starved of a blood supply. Use thin string or twine to tie around the base of the tag as tightly as you can and the skin that is being deprived of blood (which it needs to stay alive) will very soon die and fall off.

As you might expect, this third option is going to cause a degree of discomfort or pain, but if you can tolerate that downside, it is also the most effective and quickest way of getting rid of skin tags. However, do be aware that you are 'killing' a part of your body (albeit a part of your body that you do not want), so you must exercise a degree of care using this particular strategy.

ABOUT THE AUTHOR

Elizabeth Reynolds is a dermatologist. She was born and raised in England but moved to the US to fulfill her sworn duty as a skin doctor.

Elizabeth is soon to start a family with the love of her life, Johnny.